The Simple Keto Vegetarian Cookbook

Lose Weight and Improve Health with Simple and Easy To Do Ketogenic Vegetarian Recipes

Lidia Wong

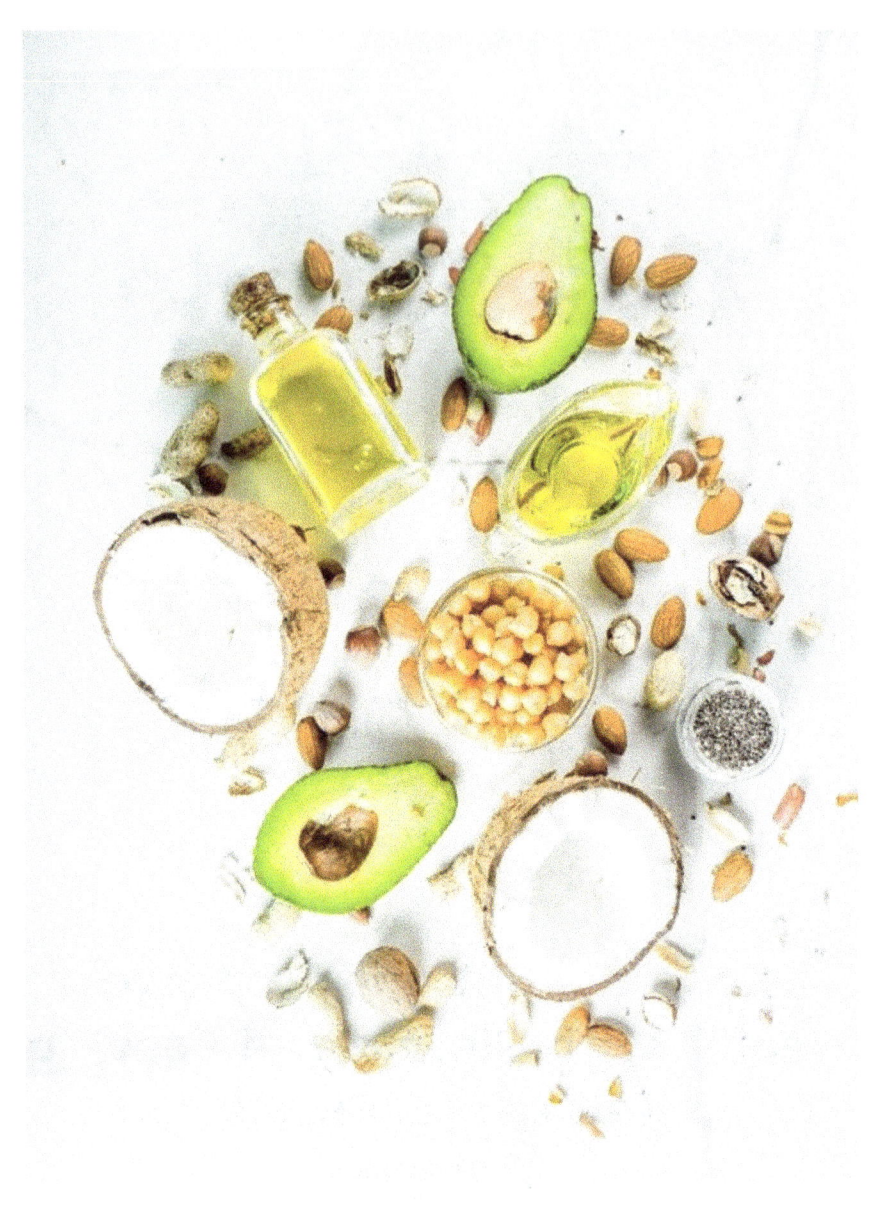

© **Copyright 2021 by Lidia Wong - All rights reserved.**

The content contained within this book may not be reproduced, duplicated or transmitted without direct written permission from the author or the publisher.
Under no circumstances will any blame or legal responsibility be held against the publisher, or author, for any damages, reparation, or monetary loss due to the information contained within this book. Either directly or indirectly.

Legal Notice:
This book is copyright protected. This book is only for personal use. You cannot amend, distribute, sell, use, quote or paraphrase any part, or the content within this book, without the consent of the author or publisher.

Disclaimer Notice:
Please note the information contained within this document is for educational and entertainment purposes only. All effort has been executed to present accurate, up to date, and reliable, complete information. No warranties of any kind are declared or implied. Readers acknowledge that the author is not engaging in the rendering of legal, financial, medical or professional advice. The content within this book has been derived from various sources. Please consult a licensed professional before attempting any techniques outlined in this book.
By reading this document, the reader agrees that under no circumstances is the author responsible for any losses, direct or indirect, which are incurred as a result of the use of information contained within this document, including, but not limited to, — errors, omissions, or inaccuracies.

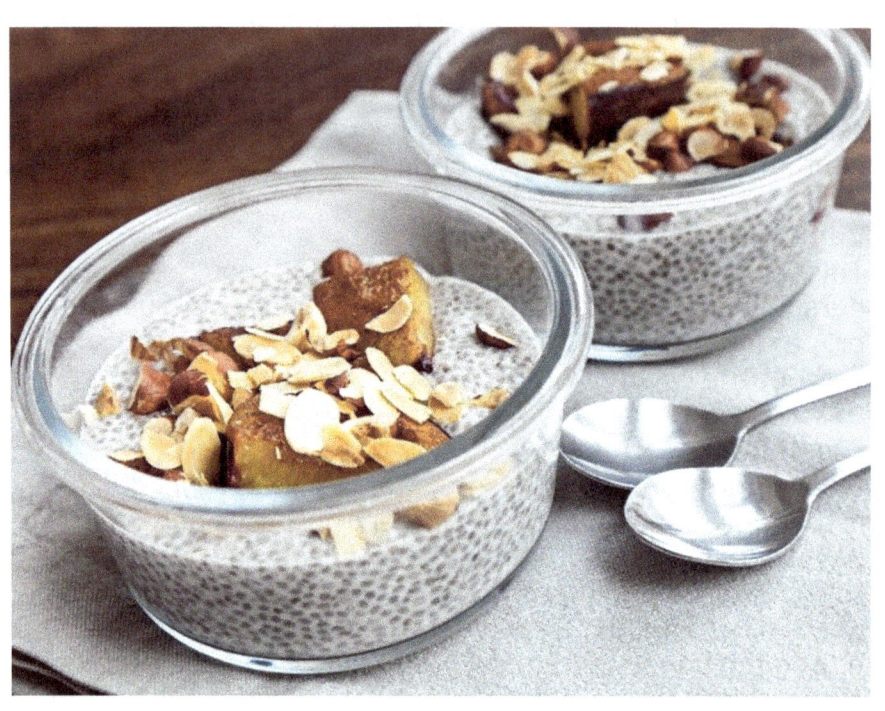

TABLE OF CONTENTS

INTRODUCTION 1

Breakfast Naan Bread 3

Avocado Ricotta Scones 5

Tomato, Green Beans and Chard Soup 7

Eggplant and Peppers Soup 9

Grilled Veggie Mix 11

Tomato and Peppers Pancakes 13

Bok Choy Salad 15

Bok Choy and Cauliflower Rice 17

Bell Peppers and Spinach Pan 19

Healthy Brussels Sprout Salad 21

Tomato Soup 22

Avocado Cilantro Tomato Salad 24

Soy Chorizo 25

Mushroom and Spinach Mix 27

Coriander Black Beans 29

Quinoa with Olives 31

Chickpeas And Veggies 33

Creamy Corn 35

Turmeric Cauliflower Rice and Tomatoes 36

Cabbage and Rice 38

Mediterranean Hummus Pizza 40

Baked Brussels Sprouts 42

Watercress Soup 44

Puréed Broccoli and Cauliflower 46

Spring Greens Soup 48

Zucchini Cream 50

Chilled Avocado-Tomato Soup 52

Soba And Green Lentil Soup 54

Thai Tofu Shirataki Stir-Fry 56

Romaine And Grape Tomato Salad With Avocado And Baby Peas 59

Italian-Style Pasta Salad 61

Indonesian-Style Potato Salad 63

Creamy Coleslaw 65

Apple-Sunflower Spinach Salad 67

Sweet Pearl Couscous Salad with Pear & Cranberries 68

Curried Tofu "Egg Salad" Pitas 70

Kale Chips 72

Savory Roasted Chickpeas 74

Garlic Tahini Spread 76

Sesame Cookies 78

Plums and Nuts Bowls 80

Vanilla Raspberries Mix 81

Orange Polenta Cake. 82

Pear Mincemeat 84

Poached Pears In Ginger Sauce. 86

Avocado Lime Dressing 87

Roasted Carrots 88

Broccoli Casserole 90

Smokey Cheddar Cheese (vegan) 92

Simple Marinara Sauce (vegan) 95

Forest Fruit Blaster (vegan) 97

Coconut Peanut Butter Fudge 99

NOTE 101

INTRODUCTION

The keto diet is the shortened term for ketogenic diet and it is essentially a high-fat and low-carb diet that helps you lose weight, thereby bringing various health benefits. This diet drastically restricts your carb intake while increasing your fat intake; this pushes your body to go into a state know as "*ketosis*". We will tackle ketosis in a bit.

The human body uses glucose from carbs to fuel metabolic pathways—meaning various bodily functions like digestion, breathing, etc.. Essentially, anything that needs energy. Even when you are resting, the body needs fuel or energy for you to continue living. If you think about it, when have you ever stopped breathing, or your heart stopped beating, or your liver stopped from cleansing the body, or your kidneys from filtering blood?

Never, unless you're dead, which is the only time in which the body doesn't need energy. In normal circumstances, glucose is the primary pathway when it comes to sourcing the body's energy.

But the body also has another pathway; it can utilize fats to fuel the various bodily processes. And this is what we call "*ketosis*". And the body can only enter ketosis when there is no glucose available, thus the reason for sticking to a low-carb diet is essential in the keto diet. Since no glucose is available, the body is pushed to use fats—it can either come from the food you consume or from your body's fat reserves—the adipose tissue or from the flabby parts of your body. This is how the keto diet helps you lose weight, by burning up all those stored fats that you have and using it to fuel bodily processes.

That said, if for whatever reason you are a vegetarian, following a ketogenic diet can be extremely difficult. A vegetarian diet is largely free of animal products, which means that food tends to be usually high in carbohydrates. Still, with careful planning, it is possible. This Cookbook will provide you with various easy and delicious dishes to help you stick to your ketogenic diet plan while being a vegetarian.

Enjoy!

Breakfast Naan Bread

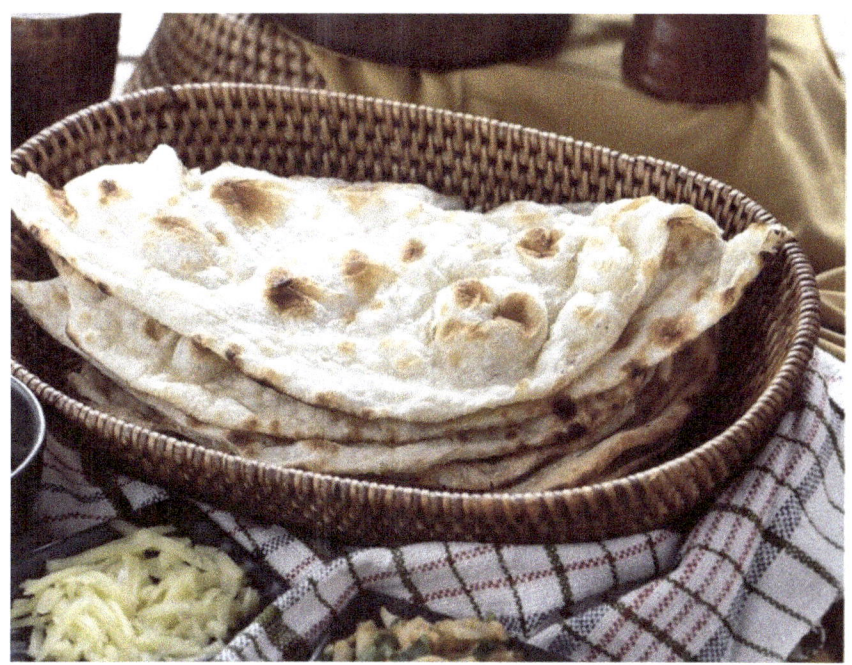

Preparation Time: 5 minutes

Cooking Time: 20 minutes

Serving: 6

Ingredients:

- ¾ cup almond flour
- 1 tsp salt + extra for sprinkling
- 2 tbsp psyllium husk powder

- 1/3 cup olive oil
- ½ tsp baking powder
- 2 cups boiling water
- Butter, for frying

Directions:

1. In a bowl, mix the almond flour, ½ teaspoon of salt, baking powder, and psyllium husk powder.
2. Mix in some olive oil and boiling water until thick batter forms. Stir thoroughly and allow the dough rising for 5 minutes.
3. Divide the dough into 6 to 8 pieces and mold it into balls. Place the balls on a parchment paper and flatten with your hands.
4. After, melt the butter in a frying pan and fry the naan on both sides until golden color.
5. Transfer the naan to a plate and use warm for breakfast.

Nutrition:

Calories:263, Total Fat:25.2 g, Saturated Fat: 6.4g, Total Carbs:3 g, Dietary Fiber: 1g, Sugar:2 g, Protein:7 g, Sodium: 376mg

Avocado Ricotta Scones

Preparation Time: 8 minutes

Cooking time: 25 minutes

Serving: 4

Ingredients:

- 2 cups almond flour
- 1 cup crumbled ricotta cheese
- 1 ripe avocado, pitted and mashed
- 3 tsp baking powder
- ½ cup butter, cold
- 1 large egg
- 1/3 cup coconut cream

Directions:

1. Preheat the oven to 350 °F and line a baking sheet with parchment paper.
2. In a large bowl, combine the almond flour and baking powder. Add the butter and mix with your hands. Top with the ricotta cheese, avocado, and combine again.
3. Lightly whisk the egg with the coconut cream

and slowly stir in the mixture using a fork. Mold 8 to 10 scones out to the batter.
4. Place the scones on the baking sheet and bake in the oven for 20 to 25 minutes or until the scones turn a golden color.
5. Remove; allow cooling for 5 minutes, and serve.

Nutrition:

Calories: 151, Total Fat: 13.2g, Saturated Fat:6.8 g, Total Carbs: 2 g, Dietary Fiber: 0g, Sugar: 2g, Protein:6 g, Sodium: 126mg

Tomato, Green Beans and Chard Soup

Preparation time: 10 minutes

Cooking time: 35 minutes

Servings: 4

Ingredients:

- 2 scallions, chopped
- 1 cup Swiss chard, chopped
- 1 tablespoon olive oil
- 1 red bell pepper, chopped
- 1 cup green beans, chopped
- 1 cup tomatoes, cubed
- 6 cups vegetable stock
- 2 tablespoons tomato passata
- Salt and black pepper to the taste
- 2 garlic cloves, minced
- 2 teaspoons thyme, chopped
- ½ teaspoon red pepper flakes

Directions:

1. Heat up a pot with the oil over medium heat, add the scallions, garlic and the pepper flakes and sauté for 5 minutes.
2. Add the chard and the other ingredients, toss, bring to a simmer and cook over medium heat for 30 minutes more.
3. Ladle the soup into bowls and serve for lunch.

Nutrition:

Calories 150, fat 8, fiber 2, carbs 4, protein 9

Eggplant and Peppers Soup

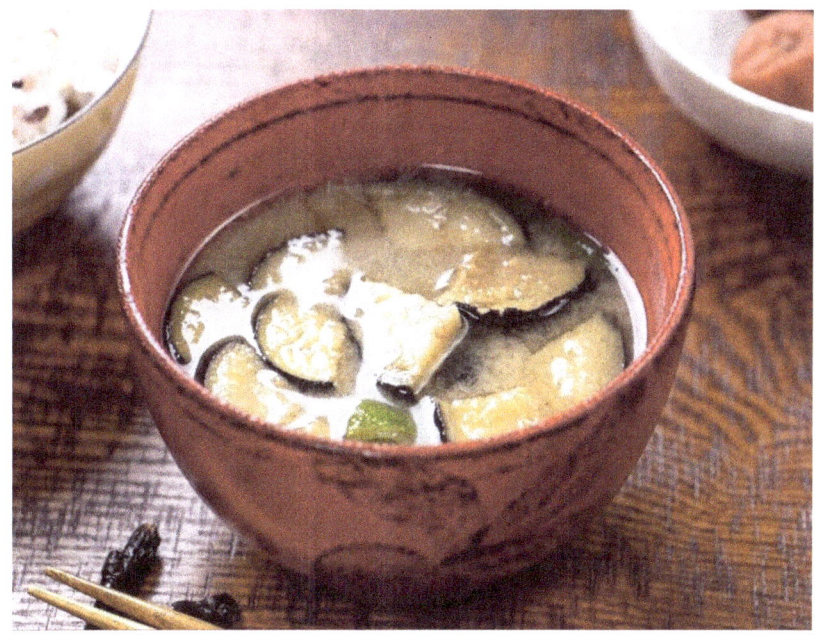

Preparation time: 10 minutes

Cooking time: 40 minutes

Servings: 4

Ingredients:

- 2 red bell peppers, chopped
- 3 scallions, chopped
- 3 garlic cloves, minced

- 2 tablespoon olive oil
- 1 bay leaf
- ½ cup coconut cream
- 1 pound eggplants, roughly cubed
- Salt and black pepper to the taste
- 5 cups vegetable stock
- 2 tablespoons basil, chopped

Directions:

1. Heat up a pot with the oil over medium heat, add the scallions and the garlic and sauté for 5 minutes.
2. Add the peppers and the eggplants and sauté for 5 minutes more.
3. Add the remaining ingredients, toss, bring to a simmer, cook for 30 minutes, ladle into bowls and serve for lunch.

Nutrition:

Calories 180, fat 2, fiber 3, carbs 5, protein 10

Grilled Veggie Mix

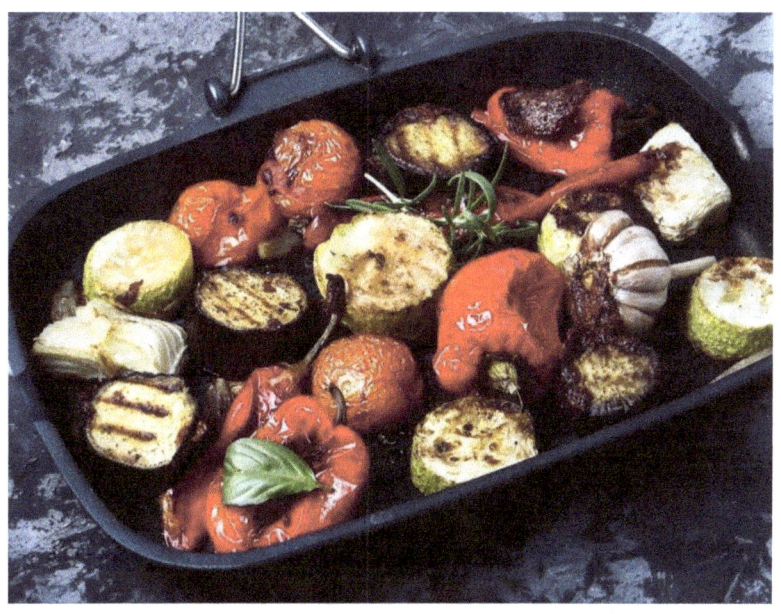

Preparation time: 10 minutes

Cooking time: 30 minutes

Servings: 4

Ingredients:

- 2 eggplants, roughly cubed
- 2 cups radishes, halved
- 1 pound cherry tomatoes, halved
- 2 green bell peppers, halved, deseeded

- 1 teaspoon chili powder
- 1 teaspoon rosemary, dried
- 1/4 cup balsamic vinegar
- Salt and black pepper to the taste
- 2 tablespoons olive oil
- 1 tablespoon basil, chopped

Directions:

1. In a bowl, combine the tomatoes with the eggplants and the other ingredients except for the basil and toss well.
2. Arrange the veggies on your preheated grill and cook over medium heat for 15 minutes on each side.
3. Divide the veggies between plates, sprinkle the basil on top and serve.

Nutrition:

Calories 120, fat 1, fiber 3, carbs 9, protein 2

Tomato and Peppers Pancakes

Preparation time: 10 minutes

Cooking time: 10 minutes

Servings: 4

Ingredients:

- 3 scallions, chopped
- 1 pound tomatoes, crushed
- 1 green bell pepper, chopped
- 1 red bell pepper, chopped
- Salt and black pepper to the taste
- 1 teaspoon coriander, ground
- 2 tablespoons almond flour
- 3 tablespoons coconut oil, melted
- 2 tablespoons flaxseed mixed with 3 tablespoons water

Directions:

1. In a bowl, combine the tomatoes with the peppers and the other ingredients except 1 tablespoon oil and stir really well.

2. Heat up a pan with the remaining oil over medium heat, add ¼ of the batter, spread into the pan, cook for 3 minutes on each side and transfer to a plate.
3. Repeat this with the rest of the batter, transfer all pancakes to a platter and serve.

Nutrition:

Calories 70, fat 2, fiber 3, carbs 10, protein 4

Bok Choy Salad

Preparation time: 10 minutes

Cooking time: 20 minutes

Servings: 4

Ingredients:

- 4 scallions, chopped
- 2 tablespoons balsamic vinegar
- 1 tablespoon chili powder
- 1 pound bok choy, torn
- 2 tablespoons olive oil
- ½ cup veggie stock
- 1 cup cherry tomatoes, halved
- 1 tablespoon garlic powder
- ¼ cup chives, chopped
- 1 teaspoon rosemary, dried
- 1 tablespoon thyme, chopped
- A pinch of sea salt and black pepper

Directions:

1. Heat up a pan with the oil over medium heat, add the scallions, garlic powder and rosemary, stir and cook for 5 minutes.
2. Add the bok choy and the rest of the ingredients, toss, cook over medium heat for 15 minutes, divide between plates and serve.

Nutrition:

Calories 107, fat 8.4, fiber 3.4, carbs 9, protein 3.1

Bok Choy and Cauliflower Rice

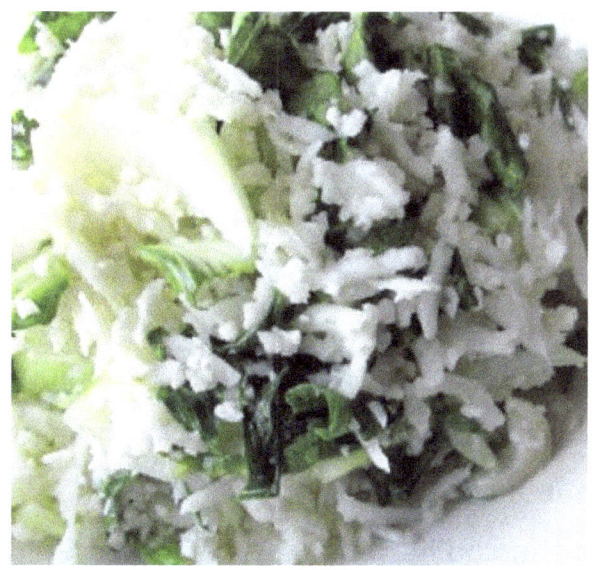

Preparation time: 10 minutes

Cooking time: 20 minutes

Servings: 4

Ingredients:

- 2 tablespoons olive oil
- 4 scallions, chopped
- 2 garlic cloves, minced
- 2 cups cauliflower rice

- ½ cup cherry tomatoes, halved
- 1 cup bok choy, torn
- 2 tablespoons thyme, chopped
- 1 tablespoon lemon juice
- Zest of ½ lemon, grated
- A pinch of sea salt and black pepper

Directions:

1. Heat up a pan with the oil over medium heat, add the scallions and the garlic and sauté for 5 minutes.
2. Add the cauliflower rice and the other ingredients, toss, cook over medium heat for 15 minutes more, divide into bowls and serve.

Nutrition:

Calories 130, fat 2, fiber 2, carbs 6, protein 8

Bell Peppers and Spinach Pan

Preparation time: 10 minutes

Cooking time: 12 minutes

Servings: 4

Ingredients:

- 1 tablespoon olive oil
- 1 red bell pepper, cut into strips
- 1 orange bell pepper, cut into strips
- 1 green bell pepper, cut into strips
- 2 cups baby spinach
- 3 garlic cloves, minced
- 2 teaspoons garlic powder
- A pinch of sea salt and black pepper
- 1 teaspoon fennel seeds, crushed
- 1 teaspoon chili powder

Directions:

1. Heat up a pan with the oil over medium high heat, add the peppers and the garlic and sauté for 2 minutes.

2. Add the spinach and the other ingredients, toss, cook over medium heat for 10 minutes more, divide between plates and serve.

Nutrition:

Calories 125, fat 3, fiber 5, carbs 9, protein 12

Healthy Brussels Sprout Salad

Preparation Time: 15 minutes

Servings: 1

Ingredients:

- 6 Brussels sprouts, washed, sliced
- ½ teaspoon apple cider vinegar
- 1 tablespoon Parmesan cheese, fresh, grated
- 1 teaspoon extra-virgin olive oil
- ¼ teaspoon pepper
- ¼ teaspoon sea salt

Directions:

1. Add all your ingredients into a large salad bowl, toss to blend. Serve and enjoy!

Nutritional Values (Per Serving):

Calories: 156 Fat: 9.6 g Carbohydrates: 10.7 g Sugar: 2.5 g Cholesterol: 10 mg Protein: 10

Tomato Soup

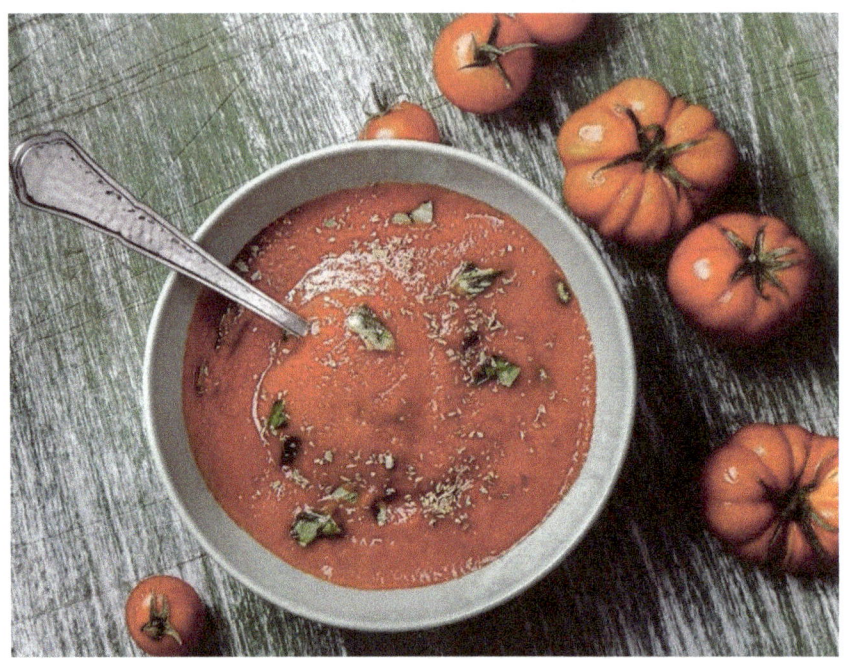

Preparation Time: 10 minutes

Cooking Time: 20 minutes

Servings: 4

Ingredients:

- 2 tablespoons tomato paste
- 1 cup onion, chopped
- 1 tablespoon extra-virgin olive oil

- 1 tablespoon garlic, minced
- 4 cups vegetable broth, low-sodium
- ½ teaspoon thyme, chopped, fresh
- 1 tablespoon basil, fresh, chopped
- 1 teaspoon oregano, fresh, chopped
- 1 cup red bell pepper, chopped
- 3 cups tomatoes, peeled, seeded, chopped
- ¼ teaspoon pepper

Directions:

1. In the saucepan, heat your oil over medium heat. Add bell pepper, garlic, onion, and tomatoes, sauté for 10 minutes. Add remaining ingredients and stir to combine. Increase the heat to high and bring to a boil. Reduce heat to low and place a lid on the pan and simmer for 10 minutes. Remove from heat. Puree the soup using a blender until smooth. Serve and enjoy!

Nutritional Values (Per Serving):

Calories: 125 Cholesterol: 0 mg Protein: 7.2 g Sugar: 8 g Carbohydrates: 13.7 g Fat: 5.4 g

Avocado Cilantro Tomato Salad

Preparation Time: 15 minutes

Servings: 4

Ingredients:

- 4 cups cherry tomatoes, halved
- 2 avocados, diced
- ¼ cup cilantro, fresh, chopped
- Juice of 1 lime, fresh
- 1 tablespoon extra-virgin olive oil
- Pepper and salt to taste

Directions:

1. In a mixing bowl add tomatoes, avocado, and cilantro. In a small bowl, combine lime juice, olive oil, pepper, and salt. Pour lime juice mixture over salad and mix well. Enjoy!

Nutritional Values (Per Serving):

Calories: 270 Fat: 23.5 g Cholesterol: 0 mg Sugar: 5.4 g Carbohydrates: 16.6 g Protein: 3.6 g

Soy Chorizo

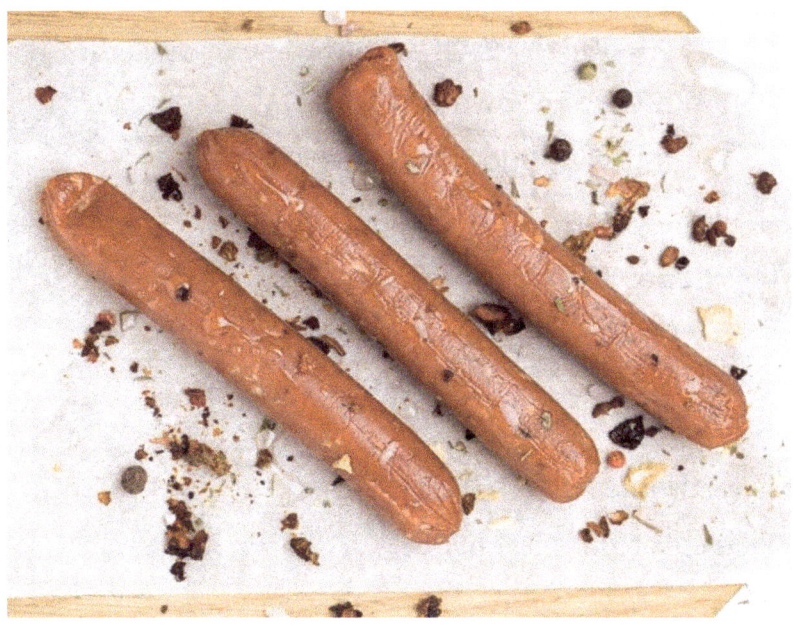

Preparation Time: 5 min

Cooking Time: 15 min

Serves: 6

Ingredients:

- 500 grams Firm Tofu, pressed and drained
- ¼ cup Red Wine Vinegar
- ¼ cup Soy Sauce
- ¼ cup Tomato Paste

- 1 tsp Paprika
- 1 tsp Chili Powder
- ½ tsp Onion Powder
- 1 tsp Garlic Powder
- 1 tsp Cumin Powder
- ½ tsp Black Pepper
- ½ tsp Salt
- ¼ cup Olive Oil

Directions:

1. Crumble tofu in a bowl. Mix in all ingredients except for the olive oil.
2. Heat olive oil in a non-stick pan.
3. Add tofu mix and stir for 10-15 minutes.
4. Serve in tacos, wraps, burritos, or rice bowls.

Nutritional Values:

Kcal per serve: 249 Fat: 18 g. Protein: 14 g. Carbs: 9 g.

Mushroom and Spinach Mix

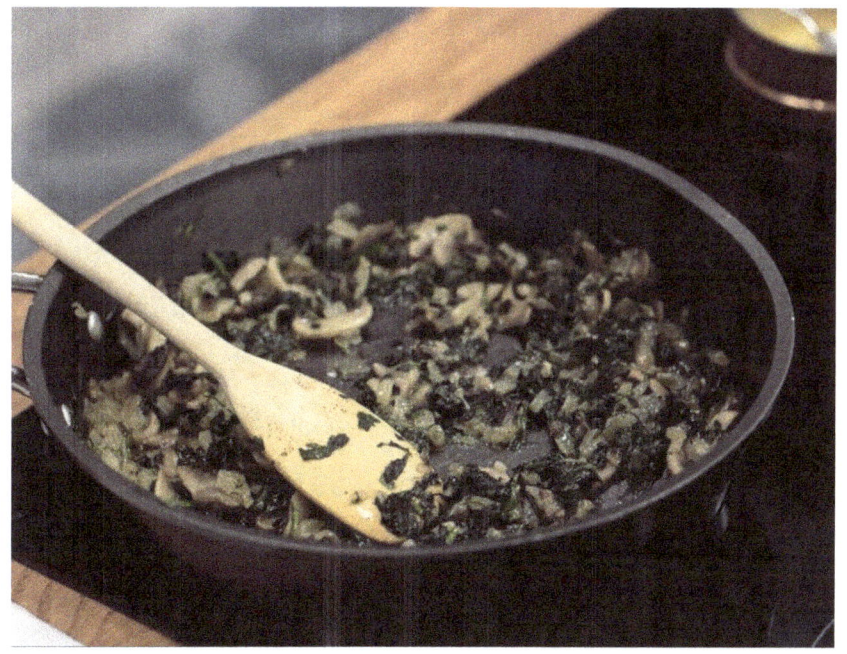

Preparation time: 10 minutes

Cooking time: 15 minutes

Servings: 4

Ingredients:

- 3 cups baby spinach
- 1 cup white mushrooms, sliced
- 2 tablespoons olive oil

- 2 tablespoons garlic, minced
- Salt and black pepper to the taste
- 2 tablespoons pine nuts, toasted
- 1 tablespoon walnuts, chopped

Directions:

1. Heat up a pan with the oil over medium heat, add the garlic, pine nuts and the walnuts and cook for 5 minutes.
2. Add the mushrooms and the other ingredients, toss, cook over medium heat for 10 minutes, divide between plates and serve.

Nutrition:

Calories 116, fat 11.3, fiber 1.1, carbs 3.5, protein 2.5

Coriander Black Beans

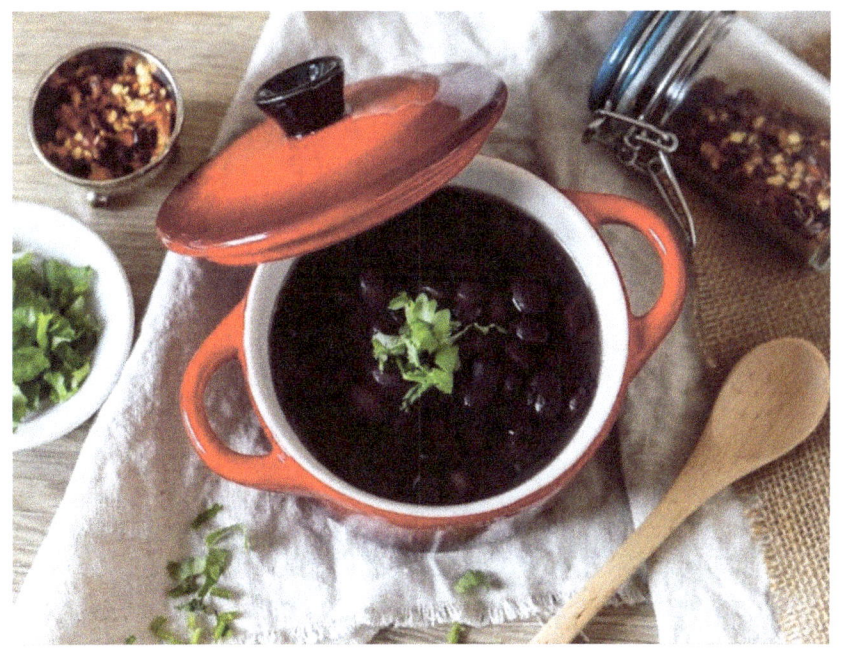

Preparation time: 10 minutes

Cooking time: 20 minutes

Servings: 4

Ingredients:

- 1 tablespoon olive oil
- 1 green bell pepper, chopped
- 2 cups canned black beans, drained and rinsed

- 1 yellow onion, chopped
- 4 garlic cloves, minced
- 1 teaspoon cumin, ground
- ½ cup chicken stock
- 1 tablespoon coriander, chopped
- A pinch of salt and black pepper

Directions:

1. Heat up a pan with the oil over medium heat, add the onion and the garlic and sauté for 5 minutes.
2. Add the black beans and the other ingredients, toss, cook over medium heat for 15 minutes more, divide between plates and serve.

Nutrition:

Calories 221, fat 5, fiber 4, carbs 9, protein 11

Quinoa with Olives

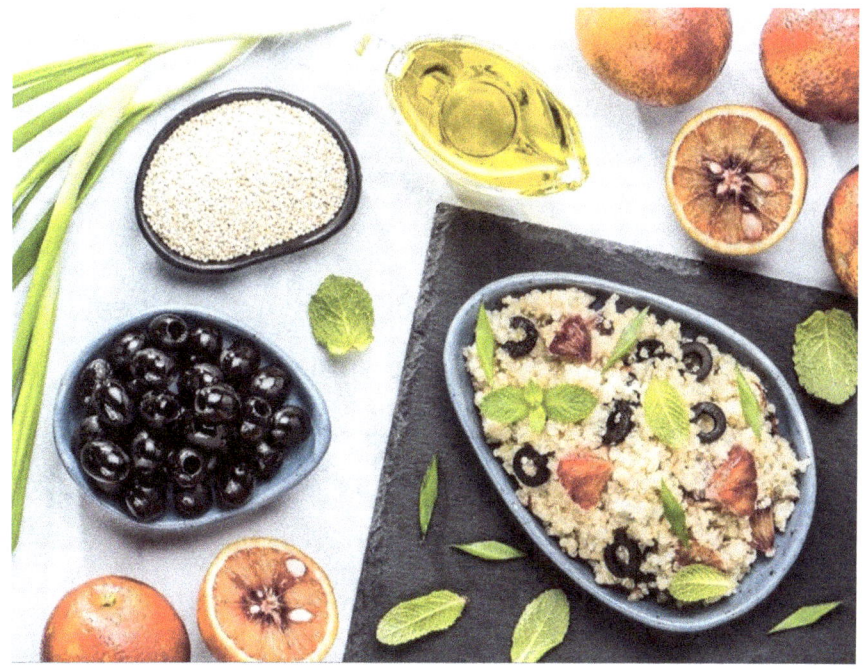

Preparation time: 10 minutes

Cooking time: 30 minutes

Servings: 4

Ingredients:

- 1 yellow onion, chopped
- 1 cup quinoa
- 1 tablespoon olive oil

- 3 cups vegetable stock
- ½ cup black olives, pitted and halved
- 2 green onions, chopped
- 2 tablespoons coconut aminos
- 1 teaspoon rosemary, dried

Directions:

1. Heat up a pot with the oil over medium heat, add the yellow onion and sauté for 5 minutes.
2. Add the quinoa and the other ingredients except for the green onions, stir, bring to a simmer and cook over medium heat for 25 minutes.
3. Divide the mix between plates, sprinkle the green onions on top and serve.

Nutrition:

Calories 261, fat 6, fiber 8, carbs 10, protein 6

Chickpeas And Veggies

Preparation time: 10 minutes

Cooking time: 8 hours

Servings: 6

Ingredients:

- 30 ounces canned chickpeas, drained
- 2 tablespoons olive oil
- 2 tablespoons rosemary, chopped
- A pinch of salt and black pepper
- 1 cup corn
- 2 cups cherry tomatoes, halved
- 2 garlic cloves, minced
- 28 ounces veggie stock
- 1 pound baby potatoes, peeled and halved
- 12 small baby carrots, peeled
- 1 yellow onion, cut into medium wedges
- 4 cups baby spinach
- 8 ounces zucchini, sliced

Directions:

1. In your slow cooker, mix chickpeas with oil, rosemary, salt, pepper, cherry tomatoes, garlic, corn, baby potatoes, baby carrots, onion, zucchini, spinach and stock, stir, cover and cook on Low for 8 hours.
2. Divide everything between plates and serve as a side dish.
3. Enjoy!

Nutrition:

Calories 273, fat 7, fiber 11, carbs 38, protein 12

Creamy Corn

Preparation time: 10 minutes

Cooking time: 3 hours

Servings: 6

Ingredients:

- 50 ounces corn
- 1 cup almond milk
- 8 ounces coconut cream
- 1 tablespoon stevia
- A pinch of white pepper

Directions:

1. In your slow cooker, mix corn with almond milk, stevia, cream and white pepper, toss, cover and cook on High for 3 hours.
2. Divide between plates and serve as a side dish.
3. Enjoy!

Nutrition:

Calories 200, fat 5, fiber 7, carbs 12, protein 4

Turmeric Cauliflower Rice and Tomatoes

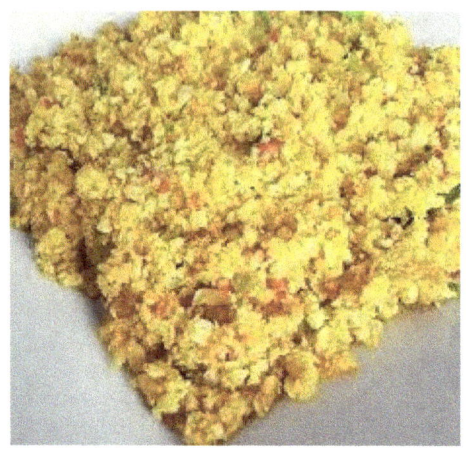

Preparation time: 10 minutes

Cooking time: 25 minutes

Servings: 4

Ingredients:

- 2 tablespoons olive oil
- 2 scallions, chopped
- 2 cups cauliflower rice
- 2 garlic cloves, minced
- 1 cup cherry tomatoes, halved

- 1 teaspoon basil, dried
- 1 teaspoon oregano, dried
- 1 cup vegetable stock
- A pinch of salt and black pepper
- ¼ teaspoon turmeric powder
- A handful of cilantro, chopped

Directions:

1. Heat up a pan with the oil over medium heat, add the scallions, garlic, basil, oregano and turmeric and sauté for 5 minutes.
2. Add the cauliflower rice, tomatoes and the remaining ingredients, toss, cook over medium heat for 20 minutes, divide between plates and serve as a side dish.

Nutrition:

Calories 77, fat 7.7, fiber 1, carbs 3.7, protein 0.7

Cabbage and Rice

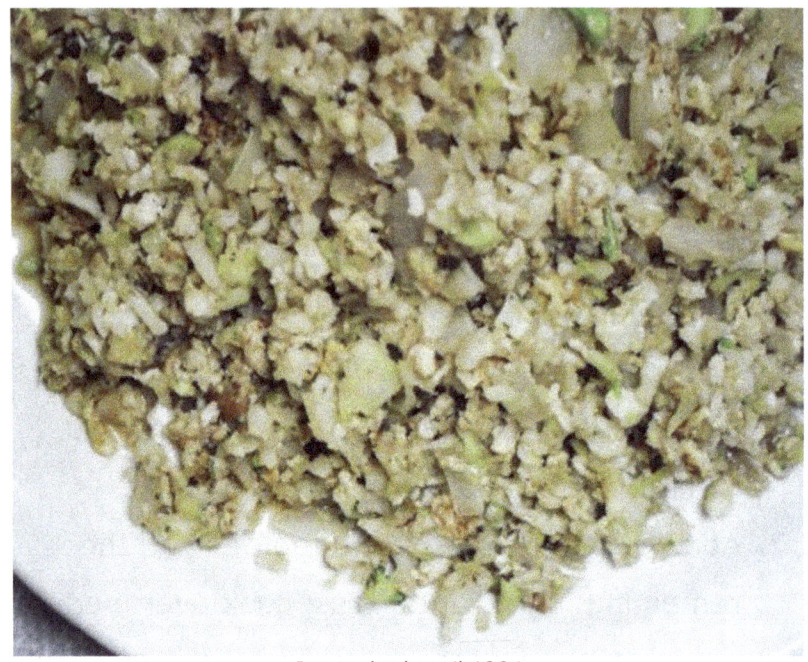

Image by larryjh1234

Preparation time: 10 minutes

Cooking time: 30 minutes

Servings: 4

Ingredients:

- 1 cup green cabbage, shredded
- 2 spring onions, chopped
- 1 cup cauliflower rice

- 2 tablespoons olive oil
- 2 tablespoons tomato passata
- 2 teaspoons balsamic vinegar
- 2 teaspoons fennel seeds, crushed
- 1 teaspoon coriander, ground
- A pinch of salt and black pepper

Directions:

1. Heat up a pan with the oil over medium heat, add the spring onions, fennel and coriander, stir and cook for 5 minutes.
2. Add the cabbage, cauliflower rice and the other ingredients, toss, cook over medium heat for 25 minutes more, divide between plates and serve.

Nutrition:

Calories 200, fat 4, fiber 1, carbs 8, protein 5

Mediterranean Hummus Pizza

Preparation time: 10 minutes

cooking time: 30 minutes

servings: 2 pizzas

Ingredients

- ½ zucchini, thinly sliced
- ½ red onion, thinly sliced
- 1 cup cherry tomatoes, halved
- 2 to 4 tablespoons pitted and chopped black olives
- Drizzle olive oil (optional
- 2 prebaked pizza crusts
- ½ cup Classic Hummus, or Roasted Red Pepper Hummus
- Pinch sea salt
- 2 to 4 tablespoons Cheesy Sprinkle

Directions

1. Preheat the oven to 400 °F. Place the zucchini, onion, cherry tomatoes, and olives in a large bowl, sprinkle them with the sea salt, and toss them a bit. Drizzle with a bit of olive oil (if using), to seal in the flavor and keep them from drying out in the oven.
2. Lay the two crusts out on a large baking sheet. Spread half the hummus on each crust, and top with the veggie mixture and some Cheesy Sprinkle. Pop the pizzas in the oven for 20 to 30 minutes, or until the veggies are soft.

Nutrition (1 pizza)

Calories: 500; Total fat: 25g; Carbs: 58g; Fiber: 12g; Protein: 19g

Baked Brussels Sprouts

Preparation time: 10 minutes

cooking time: 40 minutes

servings: 4

Ingredients

- 1 pound Brussels sprouts
- 2 teaspoons extra-virgin olive or canola oil
- 4 teaspoons minced garlic (about 4 cloves
- ½ teaspoon dried rosemary
- ½ teaspoon salt
- 1 teaspoon dried oregano
- ¼ teaspoon freshly ground black pepper
- 1 tablespoon balsamic vinegar

Directions

1. Preheat the oven to 400 ºF. Line a rimmed baking sheet with parchment paper. Trim and halve the Brussels sprouts. Transfer to a large bowl. Toss with the olive oil, garlic, oregano, rosemary, salt, and pepper to coat well.

2. Transfer to the prepared baking sheet. Bake for 35 to 40 minutes, shaking the pan occasionally to help with even browning, until crisp on the outside and tender on the inside. Remove from the oven and transfer to a large bowl. Stir in the balsamic vinegar, coating well.
3. Divide the Brussels sprouts evenly among 4 single-serving containers. Let cool before sealing the lids.

Nutrition:

Calories: 77; Fat: 3g; Protein: 4g; Carbohydrates: 12g; Fiber: 5g; Sugar: 3g; Sodium: 320mg

Watercress Soup

Preparation time: 10 minutes

Cooking time: 20 minutes

Servings: 4

Ingredients:

- 8 ounces watercress
- 1 tablespoon lemon juice
- 14 ounces veggie stock
- 1 celery stick, chopped
- A pinch of nutmeg, ground
- 4 ounces coconut milk
- A pinch of sea salt
- Black pepper to taste
- 1 onion, chopped
- 1 tablespoon olive oil
- 12 ounces sweet potatoes, peeled and chopped

Directions:

1. Heat up a large saucepan with the oil over medium heat, add onion and celery, stir and cook for 5 minutes.

2. Add sweet potato pieces and stock, stir, bring to a simmer, cover and cook on a low heat for 10 minutes.
3. Add watercress, stir, cover saucepan again and cook for 5 minutes.
4. Blend this with an immersion blender, add a pinch of nutmeg, lemon juice, salt, pepper and coconut milk, bring to a simmer again, divide into bowls and serve.
5. Enjoy!

Nutritional value/serving:

Calories 224, fat 11,8, fiber 5,7, carbs 29,6, protein 4

Puréed Broccoli and Cauliflower

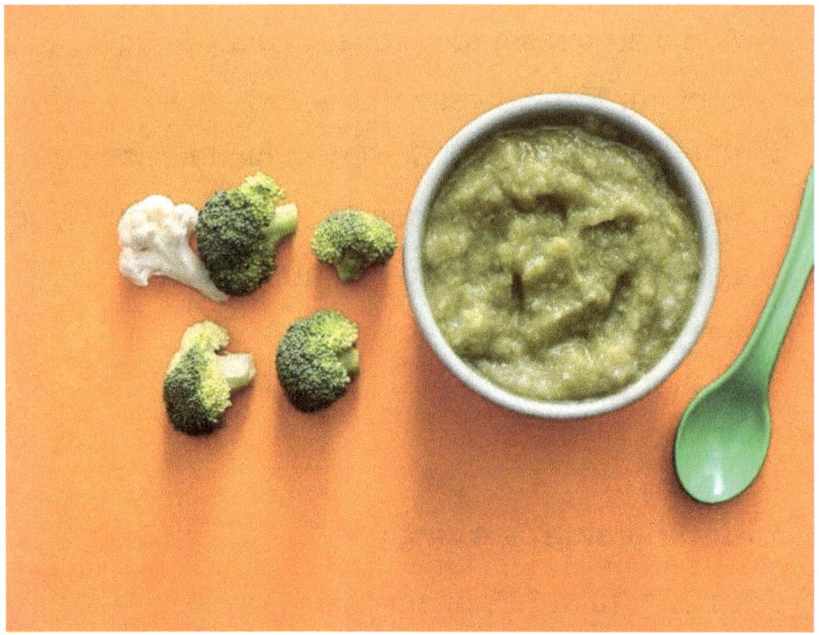

Preparation time: 10 minutes

Cooking time: 15 minutes

Servings: 5

Ingredients:

- 1 cauliflower head, separated into florets
- 1 broccoli head, separated into florets
- 2 garlic cloves, peeled and minced

- 2 bacon slices, chopped
- Salt and ground black pepper, to taste
- 2 tablespoons butter

Directions:

1. Heat up a pot with the butter over medium-high heat, add the garlic and bacon, stir, and cook for 3 minutes.
2. Add the cauliflower and broccoli florets, stir, and cook for 2 minutes. Add the water to cover them, cover the pot, and simmer for 10 minutes.
3. Add the salt and pepper, stir again, and blend soup using an immersion blender. Simmer for a couple minutes over medium heat, ladle into bowls, and serve.

Nutrition:

Calories - 230, Fat - 3, Fiber - 3, Carbs - 6, Protein - 10

Spring Greens Soup

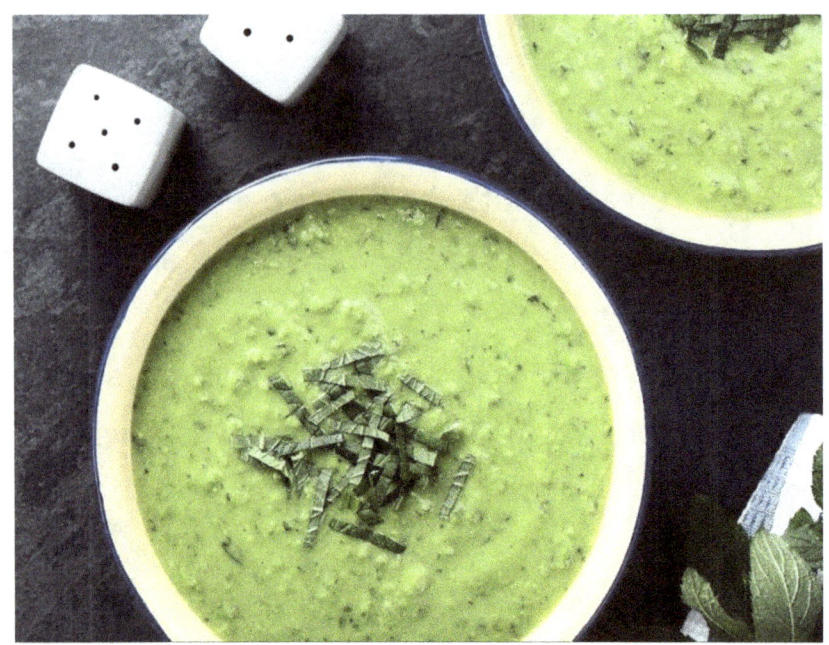

Preparation time: 10 minutes

Cooking time: 30 minutes

Servings: 4

Ingredients:

- 2 cups mustard greens, chopped
- 3 quarts vegetable stock
- 2 cups collard greens, chopped

- 1 onion, peeled and chopped
- 2 tablespoons coconut aminos
- 2 teaspoons fresh ginger, grated
- Salt and ground black pepper, to taste

Directions:

1. Put the stock into a pot, and bring to a simmer over medium-high heat.
2. Add the mustard, collard greens, onion, salt, pepper, coconut aminos, and ginger, stir, cover the pot, and cook for 30 minutes.
3. Blend the soup using an immersion blender, add more salt, and pepper, heat up over medium heat, ladle into soup bowls, and serve.

Nutrition:

Calories - 140, Fat - 2, Fiber - 1, Carbs - 3, Protein - 7

Zucchini Cream

Preparation time: 10 minutes

Cooking time: 25 minutes

Servings: 8

Ingredients:

- 6 zucchini, cut in half and sliced
- 28 ounces vegetable stock
- 1 tablespoon butter
- 1 teaspoon dried oregano
- ½ cup onion, chopped
- 3 garlic cloves, peeled and minced
- 2 ounces Parmesan cheese, grated
- Salt and ground black pepper, to taste
- ¾ cup heavy cream

Directions:

1. Heat up a pot with the butter over medium-high heat, add the onion, stir, and cook for 4 minutes.
2. Add the garlic, stir, and cook for 2 minutes.

3. Add the zucchini, stir, and cook for 3 minutes.
4. Add the stock, stir, bring to a boil, and simmer over medium heat for 15 minutes.
5. Add the oregano, salt, and pepper, stir, take off the heat, and blend using an immersion blender.
6. Heat the soup again, add the heavy cream, stir, and bring to a simmer.
7. Add the Parmesan cheese, stir, take off the heat, ladle into bowls, and serve.

Nutrition:

Calories - 160, Fat - 4, Fiber - 2, Carbs - 4, Protein - 8

Chilled Avocado-Tomato Soup

Preparation Time: 15 Minutes

Cooking Time: 0 Minutes

Servings: 4

Ingredients

- 2 garlic cloves, crushed
- 2 ripe Hass avocados
- 2 teaspoons lemon juice
- 8 fresh basil leaves, for garnish
- 2 pounds ripe plum tomatoes, coarsely chopped
- 1 (14.5-ounce) can crushed tomatoes
- 1 cup tomato juice
- Freshly ground black pepper
- Salt

Directions

1. In a blender or food processor, combine the garlic and 1/2 teaspoon of salt and process to a paste. Pit and peel one of the avocados and add it to the food processor along with the lemon juice. Process until smooth. Add the fresh and

canned tomatoes, tomato juice, and salt and pepper to taste. Process until smooth.
2. Transfer the soup to a large container, cover, and refrigerate until chilled, 2 to 3 hours.
3. Taste, adjusting seasonings if necessary. Pit and peel the remaining avocado and cut it into a small dice. Slice the basil leaves into thin strips. Ladle the soup into bowls, add the diced avocado, garnish with basil, and serve.

Soba And Green Lentil Soup

Preparation Time: 5 Minutes

Cooking Time: 55 Minutes

Servings: 4 To 6

Ingredients

- 2 tablespoons olive oil
- 1 medium onion, minced
- 1 medium carrot, halved lengthwise and sliced diagonally
- 4 ounces soba noodles, broken into thirds
- 2 garlic cloves, minced
- 1 (28-ounce) can crushed tomatoes
- 1 cup green (French) lentils, picked over, rinsed, and drained
- 1 teaspoon dried thyme
- 6 cups vegetable broth, homemade (see Light Vegetable Broth) or store-bought, or water
- Salt and freshly ground black pepper

Directions

1. In a large soup pot over medium heat, heat the oil. Add the onion, carrot, and garlic. Cover and cook until softened, about 7 minutes.
2. Uncover and stir in the tomatoes, lentils, thyme, and broth and bring to a boil.
3. Reduce heat to medium, season with salt and pepper to taste, and cover and simmer until the lentils are just tender, about 45 minutes.
4. Stir in the noodles and cook until tender, about 10 minutes longer, and serve.

Thai Tofu Shirataki Stir-Fry

Preparation Time: 35 minutes

Serving: 4

Ingredients:

For the angel hair shirataki:

- 2 (8 oz) packs angel hair shirataki

For the teriyaki tofu base:

- 2 tbsp olive oil, divided
- 1 cup sliced cremini mushrooms
- 1 ¼ lb tofu, cut into bite-size pieces
- 1 white onion, thinly sliced
- 1 red bell pepper, deseeded and sliced
- 4 garlic cloves, minced
- 1 ½ cups fresh Thai basil leaves
- Salt and black pepper to taste
- 2 tbsp toasted sesame seeds
- 1 tbsp chopped peanuts
- 1 tbsp chopped fresh scallions

For the sauce:

- 3 tbsp coconut aminos
- 2 tbsp Himalayan salt

- 1 tbsp hot sauce

Directions:

For the angel hair shirataki:

1. Boil 2 cups of water in a medium pot over medium heat.
2. Strain the shirataki pasta through a colander and rinse very well under hot running water.
3. Allow proper draining and pour the shirataki pasta into the boiling water. Cook for 3 minutes and strain again.
4. Place a dry skillet over medium heat and stir-fry the shirataki pasta until visibly dry, and makes a squeaky sound when stirred, 1 to 2 minutes. Take off the heat and set aside.

For the teriyaki tofu base:

5. Heat the olive oil in a large skillet, season the tofu with salt, black pepper, and sear in the oil on both sides until brown, 5 minutes. Transfer to a plate and set aside.
6. Add the onion, bell pepper, and mushrooms to the skillet; cook until softened, 5 minutes. Stir in the garlic and cook until fragrant, 1 minute.

7. Return the tofu to the skillet and add the pasta.
8. Quickly, combine the sauce's Ingredients in a small bowl: coconut aminos, Himalayan salt, and hot sauce. Pour the mixture over the tofu mix. Top with the Thai basil and toss well to coat. Cook for 1 to 2 minutes or until warmed through.
9. Dish the food onto serving plates and garnish with the sesame seeds, peanuts, and scallions.

Nutrition:

Calories: 598, Total Fat: 56g, Saturated Fat:18.8g, Total Carbs: 12 g, Dietary Fiber3:g, Sugar:5 g, Protein: 15g, Sodium:762 mg

Romaine And Grape Tomato Salad With Avocado And Baby Peas

Preparation time: 15 minutes

cooking time: 0 minutes

servings: 4

Ingredients

- 1 garlic clove, chopped
- 1 tablespoon chopped shallot
- 1/2 teaspoon dried basil
- 1 medium head romaine lettuce, cut into 1/4-inch strips
- 1/2 teaspoon salt
- 1/8 teaspoon freshly ground black pepper
- 1/4 teaspoon brown sugar (optional
- 3 tablespoons white wine vinegar
- 1/3 cup olive oil
- 12 ripe grape tomatoes, halved
- 1/2 cup frozen baby peas, thawed
- 8 kalamata olives, pitted
- 1 ripe Hass avocado

Directions

1. In a blender or food processor, combine the garlic, shallot, basil, salt, pepper, sugar, and vinegar until smooth. Add the oil and blend until emulsified. Set aside.
2. In a large bowl, combine the lettuce, tomatoes, peas, and olives. Pit and peel the avocado and cut into 1/2-inch dice.
3. Add to the bowl, along with enough dressing to lightly coat.
4. Toss gently to combine and serve.

Italian-Style Pasta Salad

Preparation time: 5 minutes

cooking time: 10 minutes

servings: 4 to 6

Ingredients

- 8 ounces penne, rotini, or other small pasta
- 1 1/2 cups cooked or 1 (15.5-ouncecan chickpeas, drained and rinsed
- 1/2 cup pitted kalamata olives
- 1/2 cup frozen peas, thawed
- 1/2 cup minced oil-packed sun-dried tomatoes
- 1 (6-ouncejar marinated artichoke hearts, drained
- 2 jarred roasted red peppers, chopped
- 1 tablespoon capers
- 2 teaspoons dried chives
- 1/2 cup olive oil
- 1/4 cup white wine vinegar
- 1/2 teaspoon dried basil
- 1 garlic clove, minced
- Salt and freshly ground black pepper

Directions

1. In a pot of boiling salted water, cook the pasta, occasionally stirring, until al dente, about 10 minutes. Drain well and transfer to a large bowl. Add the chickpeas, olives, tomatoes, artichoke hearts, roasted peppers, peas, capers, and chives. Toss gently and set aside.
2. In a small bowl, combine the oil, vinegar, basil, garlic, sugar, and salt and black pepper to taste. Pour the dressing onto the pasta salad and toss to combine. Serve chilled or at room temperature.

Indonesian-Style Potato Salad

Preparation time: 10 minutes

cooking time: 30 minutes

servings: 4 to 6

Ingredients

- 1 1/2 pounds small white potatoes, unpeeled
- 4 green onions, chopped
- 1 cup frozen peas, thawed
- 1/2 cup shredded carrot
- 1 tablespoon grapeseed oil
- 1 garlic clove, minced
- 1/2 teaspoon Asian chili paste
- 1/3 cup creamy peanut butter
- 2 tablespoons soy sauce
- 1 tablespoon rice vinegar
- ¾ cup unsweetened coconut milk
- 3 tablespoons chopped unsalted roasted peanuts, for garnish

Directions

1. In a large pot of boiling salted water, cook the potatoes until tender, 20 to 30 minutes. Drain well and set aside to cool.
2. When cool enough to handle, cut the potatoes into 1-inch chunks and transfer to a large bowl. Add the peas, carrot, and green onions, and set aside.
3. In a small saucepan, heat the oil over medium heat. Add the garlic and cook until fragrant, about 30 seconds. Stir in the peanut butter, chili paste, soy sauce, vinegar, and about half of the coconut milk. Simmer over medium heat for 5 minutes, frequently stirring to make a smooth sauce. Add as much of the remaining coconut milk as needed for a creamy consistency. Pour the dressing over the salad and toss well to combine. Garnish with peanuts and serve.

Creamy Coleslaw

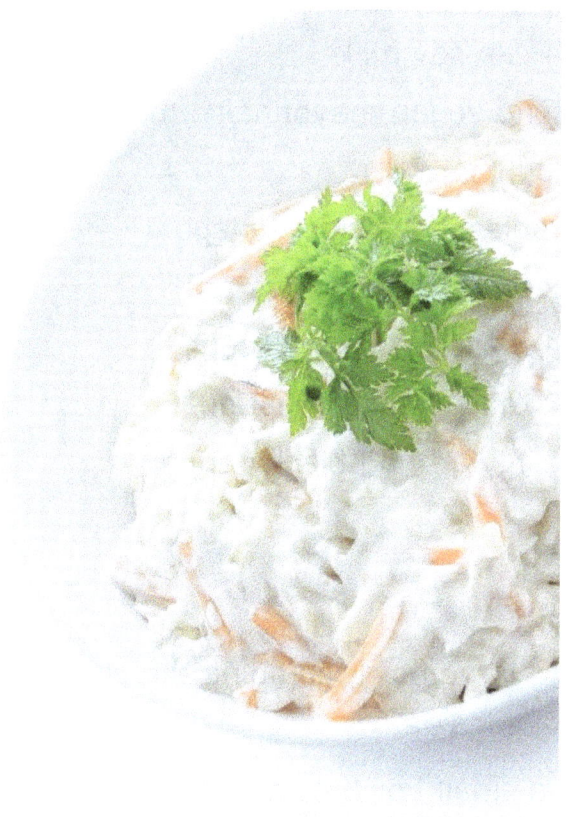

Preparation time: 10 minutes

cooking time: 0 minutes

servings: 4

Ingredients

- 1 small head green cabbage, finely shredded
- 1 large carrot, shredded
- 1/4 cup soy milk
- ¾ cup vegan mayonnaise, homemade or store-bought
- 2 tablespoons cider vinegar
- 1/2 teaspoon dry mustard
- 1/4 teaspoon celery seeds
- 1/2 teaspoon salt (optional
- Freshly ground black pepper

Directions

1. In a large bowl, combine the cabbage and carrot and set aside.
2. In a small bowl, combine the mayonnaise, soy milk, vinegar, mustard, celery seeds, salt, and pepper to taste. Mix until smooth and well blended. Add the dressing to the slaw and mix well to combine. Taste, adjust seasonings if necessary, and serve.

Apple-Sunflower Spinach Salad

Preparation Time: 5 Minutes

Cooking Time: 0 Minutes

Servings:1

Ingredients

- 1 cup baby spinach
- ½ apple, cored and chopped
- 2 tablespoons sunflower seeds or Cinnamon-Lime Sunflower Seeds
- ¼ red onion, thinly sliced (optional)
- 2 tablespoons dried cranberries
- 2 tablespoons Raspberry Vinaigrette

Directions

1. Arrange the spinach on a plate. Top with the apple, red onion (if using), sunflower seeds, and cranberries, and drizzle with the vinaigrette.

Nutrition, per Serving

Calories: 444; Protein: 7g; Total fat: 28g; Saturated fat: 3g; Carbohydrates: 53g; Fiber: 8g

Sweet Pearl Couscous Salad with Pear & Cranberries

Preparation Time: 5 Minutes

Cooking Time: 10 Minutes

Servings: 4

Ingredients

- 1 cup pearl couscous
- 1½ cups water
- ¼ cup olive oil
- ¼ cup freshly squeezed orange juice
- 1 tablespoon sugar, maple syrup, or Simple Syrup
- Salt
- 1 pear, cored and diced
- ½ cucumber, diced
- ¼ cup dried cranberries or raisins

Directions

1. In a small pot, combine the couscous, water, and a pinch of salt. Bring to a boil over high heat, turn the heat to low, and cover the pot.

Simmer for about 10 minutes, until the couscous is al dente.

2. Meanwhile, in a large bowl, whisk together the olive oil, orange juice, and sugar. Season to taste with salt and whisk again to combine.
3. Add the pear, cucumber, cranberries, and cooked couscous. Toss to combine. Store leftovers in an airtight container in the refrigerator for up to 1 week.

Nutrition (per Serving)

Calories: 365; Protein: 6g; Total fat: 14g; Saturated fat: 2g; Carbohydrates: 55g; Fiber: 4g

Curried Tofu "Egg Salad" Pitas

Preparation time: 15 minutes

cooking time: 0 minutes

servings: 4 sandwiches

Ingredients

- 1 pound extra-firm tofu, drained and patted dry
- 1/2 cup vegan mayonnaise, homemade or store-bought
- 1/4 cup chopped mango chutney, homemade or store-bought
- 2 teaspoons Dijon mustard
- 1/8 teaspoon ground cayenne
- ¾ cup shredded carrots
- 2 celery ribs, minced
- 1 tablespoon hot or mild curry powder
- 1 teaspoon salt
- 1/4 cup minced red onion
- 8 small Boston or other soft lettuce leaves
- 4 7-inchwhole wheat pita breads, halved

Directions

1. Crumble the tofu and place it in a large bowl. Add the mayonnaise, chutney, mustard, curry powder, salt, and cayenne, and stir well until thoroughly mixed.
2. Add the carrots, celery, and onion and stir to combine. Refrigerate for 30 minutes to allow the flavors to blend.
3. Tuck a lettuce leaf inside each pita pocket, spoon some tofu mixture on top of the lettuce, and serve.

Kale Chips

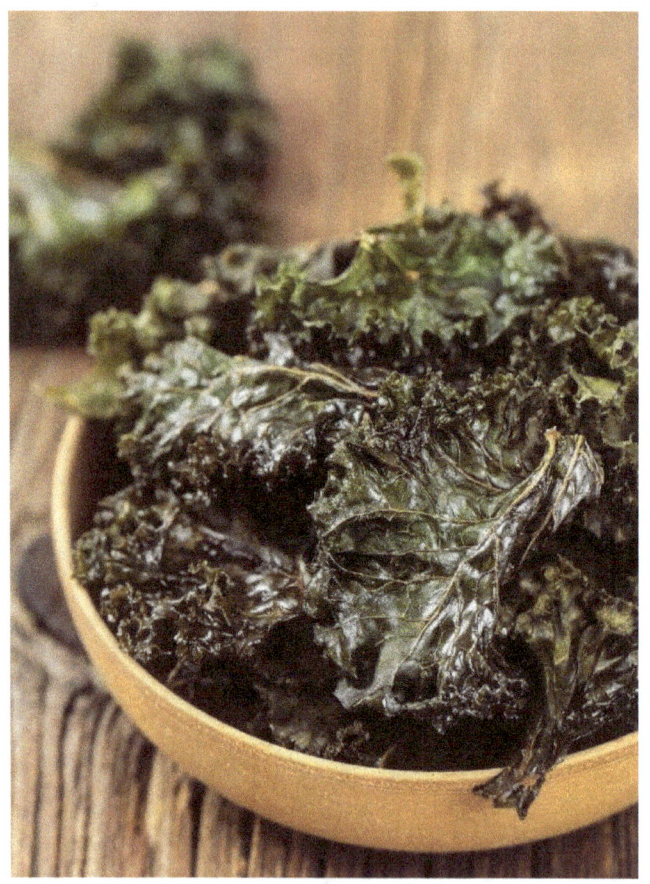

Preparation time: 5 minutes

cooking time: 25 minutes

servings: 2

Ingredients

- 1 large bunch kale
- ½ teaspoon chipotle powder
- 1 tablespoon extra-virgin olive oil
- ½ teaspoon smoked paprika
- ¼ teaspoon salt

Directions

1. Preheat the oven to 275 °F.
2. Line a large baking sheet with parchment paper. In a large bowl, stem the kale and tear it into bite-size pieces. Add the olive oil, chipotle powder, smoked paprika, and salt.
3. Toss the kale with tongs or your hands, coating each piece well.
4. Spread the kale over the parchment paper in a single layer.
5. Bake for 25 minutes, turning halfway through, until crisp.
6. Cool for 10 to 15 minutes before dividing and storing in 2 airtight containers.

Nutrition:

Calories: 144; Fat: 7g; Protein: 5g; Carbohydrates: 18g; Fiber: 3g; Sugar: 0g; Sodium: 363mg

Savory Roasted Chickpeas

Preparation time: 5 minutes

cooking time: 25 minutes

servings: 1 cup

Ingredients

- 1 (14-ouncecan chickpeas, rinsed and drained, or 1½ cups cooked
- 2 tablespoons tamari, or soy sauce
- 1 tablespoon nutritional yeast
- 1 teaspoon smoked paprika, or regular paprika
- ½ teaspoon garlic powder
- 1 teaspoon onion powder

Directions

1. Preheat the oven to 400 °F.
2. Toss the chickpeas with all the other ingredients, and spread them out on a baking sheet. Bake for 20 to 25 minutes, tossing halfway through.

3. Bake these at a lower temperature, until fully dried and crispy, if you want to keep them longer.
4. You can easily double the batch, and if you dry them out they will keep about a week in an airtight container.

Nutrition (¼ cup)

Calories: 121; Total fat: 2g; Carbs: 20g; Fiber: 6g; Protein: 8g

Garlic Tahini Spread

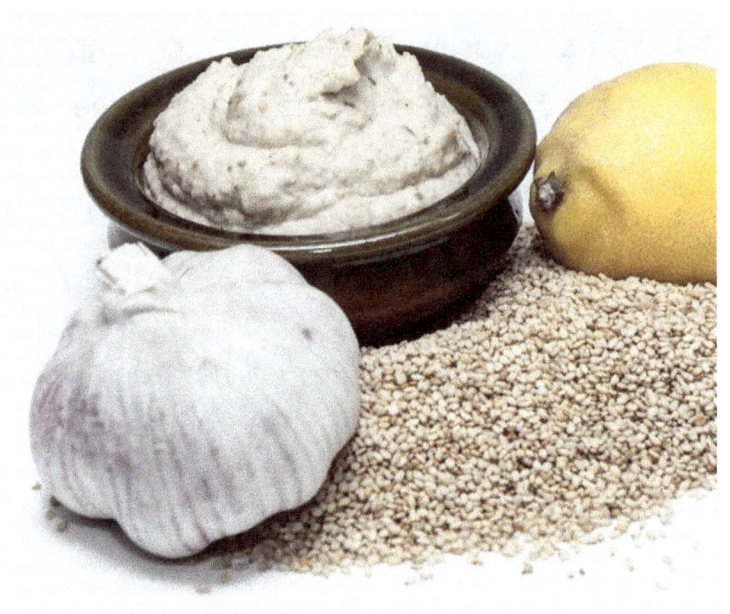

Preparation time: 10 minutes

Cooking time: 15 minutes

Servings: 4

Ingredients:

- 1 cup coconut cream
- 4 garlic cloves, minced
- 2 tablespoons tahini paste

- Juice of 1 lime
- ¼ teaspoon turmeric powder
- 1 teaspoon sweet paprika
- A pinch of salt and black pepper
- 1 tablespoon olive oil

Directions:

1. Heat up a pan with the oil over medium heat, add the garlic, turmeric and paprika and cook for 5 minutes.
2. Add the rest of the ingredients, stir, cook over medium heat for 10 minutes more, blend using an immersion blender, divide into bowls and serve.

Nutrition:

Calories 170, fat 7.3, fiber 4, carbs 1, protein 5

Sesame Cookies

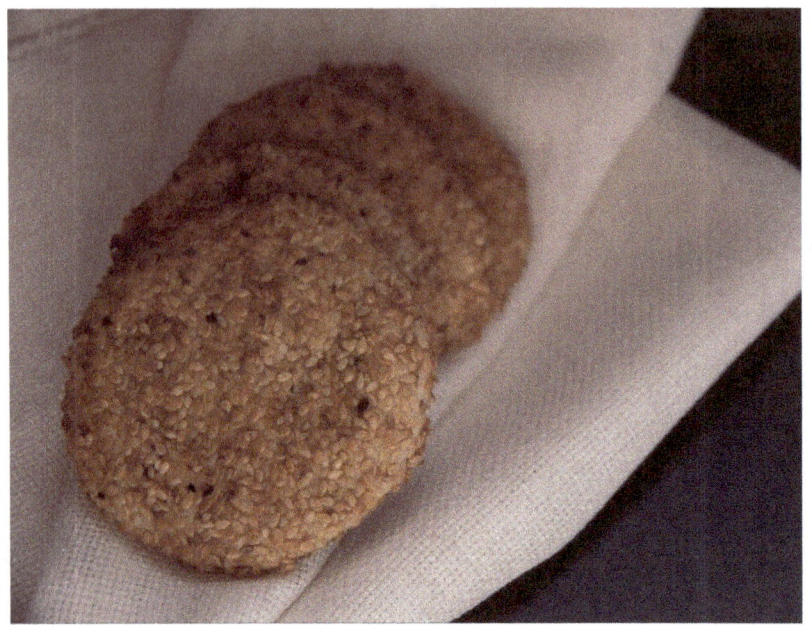

Preparation time: 15 minutes

cooking time: 0 minutes

servings: 3 dozen cookies

Ingredients

- ¾ cup vegan margarine, softened
- 1/2 cup light brown sugar
- 1 teaspoon pure vanilla extract

- 2 tablespoons pure maple syrup
- 2 cups whole-grain flour
- 1/4 teaspoon salt
- ¾ cup sesame seeds, lightly toasted

Directions

1. In a large bowl, cream together the margarine and sugar until light and fluffy. Blend in the vanilla, maple syrup, and salt. Stir in the flour and sesame seeds and mix well.
2. Roll the dough into a cylinder about 2 inches in diameter. Wrap it in plastic wrap and refrigerate for 1 hour or longer. Preheat the oven to 325 °F.
3. Slice the cookie dough into 1/8-inch-thick rounds and arrange on an ungreased baking sheet about 2 inches apart. Bake until light brown, about 12 minutes. When completely cool, store in an airtight container.

Plums and Nuts Bowls

Preparation time: 5 minutes

Cooking time: 0 minutes

Servings: 2

Ingredients:

- 2 tablespoons stevia
- 1 cup plums, pitted and halved
- 1 cup walnuts, chopped
- 1 teaspoon vanilla extract

Directions:

1. In a bowl, mix the plums with the walnuts and the other ingredients, toss, divide into 2 bowls and serve cold.

Nutrition:

Calories 400, fat 23, fiber 4, carbs 6, protein 7

Vanilla Raspberries Mix

Preparation time: 10 minutes

Cooking time: 10 minutes

Servings: 4

Ingredients:

- 1 cup water
- 1 cup raspberries
- 1 teaspoon nutmeg, ground
- 3 tablespoons stevia
- ½ teaspoon vanilla extract

Directions:

1. In a pan, combine the raspberries with the water and the other ingredients, toss, cook over medium heat for 10 minutes, divide into bowls and serve.

Nutrition:

Calories 20, fat 0.4, fiber 2.1, carbs 4, protein 0.4

Orange Polenta Cake.

Preparation Time: 30 Minutes

Servings: 6

Ingredients:

- 1¼ cups all-purpose flour
- 1 cup unsweetened almond milk
- 2/3 cup plus 1 tablespoon natural sugar
- 1 navel orange, peeled and sliced into ⅛-inch-thick rounds
- ⅓ cup fine-ground cornmeal
- ⅓ cup plus 2 tablespoons marmalade
- ¼ cup finely ground almonds
- ¼ cup vegan butter, softened
- 1½ teaspoons baking powder
- 1 teaspoon pure vanilla extract
- ¾ teaspoon salt

Directions:

1. Lightly oil a baking tray that will fit in the steamer basket of your Cooker.

2. Sprinkle a tablespoon of sugar over the base of the baking tray and top with the orange slices.
3. In a bowl combine the flour, cornmeal, baking powder, almonds, and salt.
4. In another bowl combine the remaining sugar, the butter, 1/3 cup of marmalade, and vanilla and mix well. Slowly stir in the almond milk.
5. Combine the wet and dry mixes into a smooth batter.
6. Pour the batter into your baking tray and put the tray in your steamer basket.
7. Pour the minimum amount of water into the base of your Cooker and lower the steamer basket.
8. Seal and cook on Steam for 12 minutes.
9. Release the pressure quickly and set to one side to cool a little.
10. Warm the remaining 2 tablespoons of marmalade and brush over the cake.

Pear Mincemeat.

Preparation Time: 35 Minutes

Servings: 6

Ingredients:

- 4 firm ripe Bosc pears, peeled, cored, and chopped
- 1 large orange
- 1½ cups apple juice
- 1 cup raisins (dark, golden, or a combination)
- 1¼ cups granola of your choice
- 1 cup chopped dried apples, pears, or apricots, or a combination
- ½ cup packed dark brown sugar or granulated natural sugar
- 2 tablespoons cider vinegar
- ¼ cup brandy or 1 teaspoon brandy extract
- 2 tablespoons pure maple syrup or agave nectar
- ½ teaspoon ground cinnamon
- ½ teaspoon ground allspice
- ½ teaspoon ground nutmeg
- ¼ teaspoon ground cloves

- Pinch of salt

Directions:

1. Zest the orange, then peel it, deseed it, and quarter it.
2. Blend the orange flesh and zest and put in your Cooker.
3. Add the pears, dried fruits, juice, sugar, brandy spices, vinegar, and salt.
4. Seal and cook on Stew for 12 minutes.
5. Release the pressure naturally, take out some of the juice, then reseal and cook another 12 minutes.
6. In a bowl mix the granola and syrup.
7. Release the pressure of the Cooker naturally and sprinkle the crumble on top.
8. Seal the Cooker and cook on Stew for another 5 minutes.
9. Release the pressure naturally and serve.

Poached Pears In Ginger Sauce.

Preparation Time: 25 Minutes

Servings: 6

Ingredients:

- 2½ cups white grape juice
- 6 firm ripe cooking pears, peeled, halved, and cored
- ¼ cup natural sugar, plus more if needed
- ½ cinnamon stick
- 6 strips lemon zest
- 2 teaspoons grated fresh ginger
- Juice of 1 lemon
- Pinch of salt

Directions:

1. Warm the grape juice, ginger, lemon zest, salt, and sugar until blended.
2. Add the cinnamon stick and the pears.
3. Seal and cook on Stew for 12 minutes.
4. Take the pears out.
5. Add lemon juice and more sugar to the liquid.
6. Cook with the lid off a few minutes to thicken.
7. Serve.

Avocado Lime Dressing

Preparation time: 5 minutes

Cooking time: 0 minutes

Servings: 6

Ingredients:

- 1 avocado, halved
- 1 garlic clove, peeled
- Leaves of 1 bunch fresh cilantro
- ¼ cup avocado oil
- 2 tablespoons water
- 2 tablespoons freshly squeezed lime juice
- 1 teaspoon garlic salt

Directions:

1. Combine all the ingredients in a high-powered blender or a food processor and pulse until thoroughly combined, 2 to 3 minutes. Transfer to a small mason jar and store in the refrigerator until ready to use.

Nutrition:

Calories 146, fat 14g, protein 1g, carbs 4g, fiber 2g, sugar 0g, sodium 51mg

Roasted Carrots

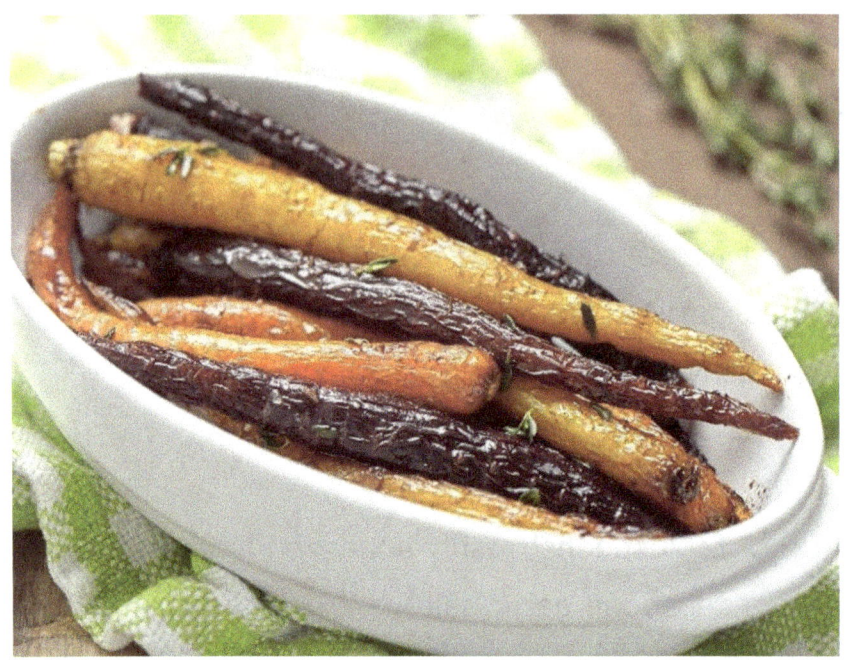

Preparation Time: 10 minutes

Cooking Time: 35 minutes

Servings: 6

Ingredients:

- 16 small carrots
- 1 tbsp dried basil
- 1 tbsp fresh parsley, chopped

- 6 garlic cloves, minced
- 4 tbsp olive oil
- 1 1/2 tsp salt

Directions:

1. Preheat the oven to 375 F/ 190 C.
2. In a bowl, combine together oil, carrots, basil, garlic, and salt.
3. Spread the carrots onto a baking tray and bake in preheated oven for 35 minutes.
4. Garnish with parsley and serve.

Nutrition:

Calories 139 Fat 9.4 g Carbohydrates 14.2 g Sugar 6.6 g Protein 1.3 g Cholesterol 0 mg

Broccoli Casserole

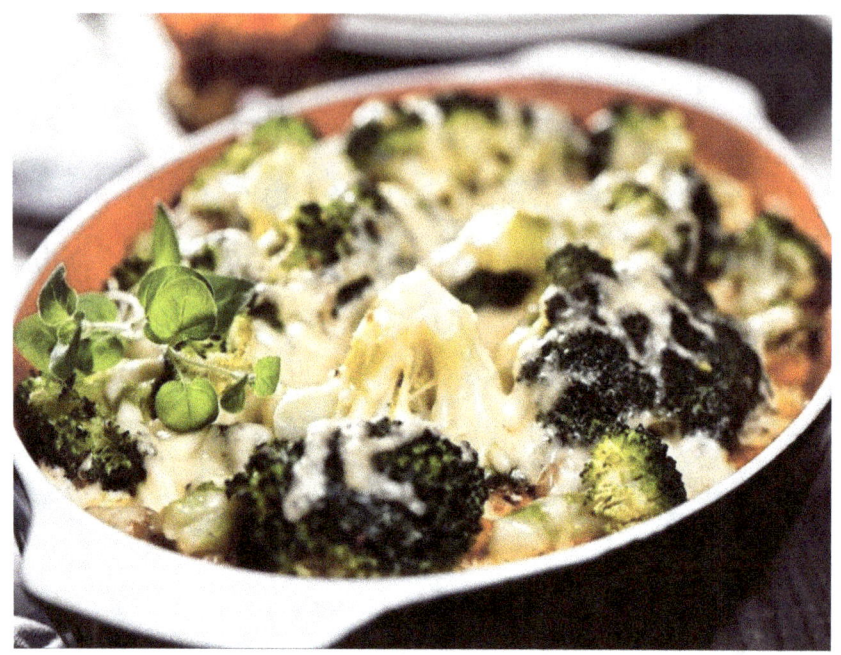

Preparation Time: 5 minutes

Cooking Time: 30 minutes

Servings: 4

Ingredients:

- 2 eggs, whisked
- 1 lb. broccoli florets
- 15 oz. coconut cream

- 1 cup parmesan, grated
- 2 cups cheddar, grated
- 1 tbsp. parsley; chopped
- 3 tbsp. ghee; melted
- 1 tbsp. mustard
- A pinch of salt and black pepper

Directions:

1. Grease a baking pan that fits the air fryer with the ghee and arrange the broccoli on the bottom.
2. Add the cream, mustard, salt, pepper and the eggs and toss
3. Sprinkle the cheese on top, put the pan in the air fryer and cook at 380°F for 30 minutes
4. Divide between plates and serve.

Nutrition:

Calories: 244 Fat: 12g Fiber: 3g Carbs: 5g Protein: 12g

Smokey Cheddar Cheese (vegan)

Preparation time: 20 minutes

Cooking time: 0 minute

Servings: 8

Ingredients:

- 1 cup raw cashews (unsalted)
- 1 cup macadamia nuts (unsalted)
- 4 tsp. tapioca starch
- ¼ cup fresh lime juice
- ½ tsp. liquid smoke
- ¼ cup tahini
- ¼ cup paprika powder
- ½ tsp. ground mustard seeds
- 2 tbsp. onion powder
- 1 tsp. Himalayan salt
- 1 cup water
- ½ tsp. chili powder
- 1 tbsp. coconut oil

Directions:

1. Cover the cashews with water in a small bowl and let sit for 4 to 6 hours. Rinse and drain the cashews after soaking. Make sure no water is left.
2. Mix the tapioca starch with the cup of water in a small saucepan. Heat the pan over medium heat.
3. Bring the water with tapioca starch to a boil. After 1 minute, take the pan off the heat and set the mixture aside to cool down.
4. Put all the remaining ingredients—except the coconut oil—in a blender or food processor. Blend until these ingredients are combined into a smooth mixture.
5. Stir in the tapioca starch with water and blend again until all ingredients have fully incorporated.
6. Grease a medium-sized bowl with the coconut oil to prevent the cheese from sticking to the edges. Gently pour the mixture into the bowl.

7. Refrigerate the bowl, uncovered, for about 3 hours until the cheese is firm and ready to enjoy!
8. Alternatively, store the cheese in an airtight container in the fridge and consume within 6 days. Store for a maximum of 60 days in the freezer and thaw at room temperature.

Nutrition:

Calories: 249 kcal, Net Carbs: 6.9g, Fat: 21.7g, Protein: 6.1g, Fiber: 4.3g, Sugar: 2.6g

Simple Marinara Sauce (vegan)

Preparation Time: 10 minutes

Cooking Time: 10 minutes

Servings: 8

Ingredients:

- 3 tbsp. olive oil
- 1 14-oz. can peeled tomatoes (no sugar added)
- ⅓ cup red onion (diced)
- 2 garlic cloves (minced)
- ½ tsp. cayenne pepper
- 2 tbsp. oregano (fresh and chopped, or 1 tbsp. dried)
- Optional: 1 tbsp. sunflower seed butter (use grass-fed butter for a lacto sauce)

Directions:

1. Heat the olive oil in a medium-sized skillet over medium heat.
2. Add the onions, garlic, salt, and cayenne pepper. Sauté the onions until translucent while stirring the ingredients.

3. Add the peeled tomatoes and more salt and pepper to taste.
4. Stir the ingredients, cover the skillet, and allow the sauce to softly cook for 10 minutes.
5. Add the oregano, and if desired, stir in the optional butter.
6. Take the skillet off the heat. The sauce is now ready to be used in a recipe!
7. Alternatively, store the sauce in an airtight container in the fridge and consume within 3 days. Store for a maximum of 30 days in the freezer and thaw at room temperature.

Nutrition:

Calories: 23kcal, Net Carbs: 2.8g, Fat: 1.1g, Protein: 0.7g, Fiber: 0.9g, Sugar: 0.1g

Forest Fruit Blaster (vegan)

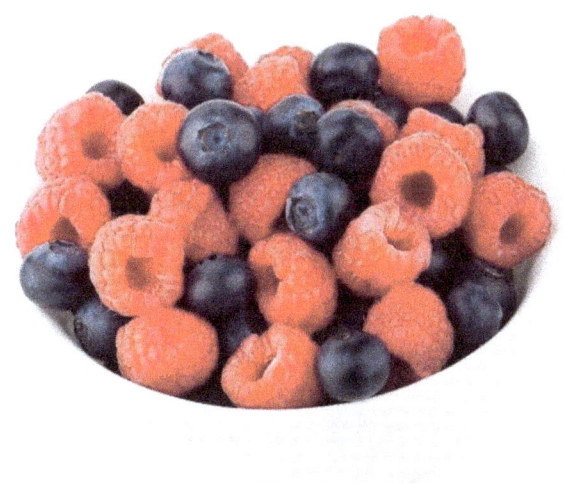

Preparation Time: 5 minutes

Cooking Time: 0 minute

Servings: 4

Ingredients:

- ¼ cup mixed berries (fresh or frozen)
- 2 cups full-fat coconut milk
- ½ kiwi (peeled)

- 2 scoops organic soy protein (vanilla flavor)
- ½ cup water
- Optional: 2 ice cubes

Directions:

1. Add all the ingredients to a blender, including the optional ice if desired, and blend for 1 minute.
2. Transfer the shake to a large cup or shaker, and enjoy!
3. Alternatively, store the smoothie in an airtight container or a mason jar, keep it in the fridge, and consume within 2 days. Store for a maximum of 30 days in the freezer and thaw at room temperature.

Nutrition:

Calories: 275kcal, Fat:24.8g, Protein: 8.5g, Net carbs: 4g, Fiber: 1.9g, Sugar: 3.4g

Coconut Peanut Butter Fudge

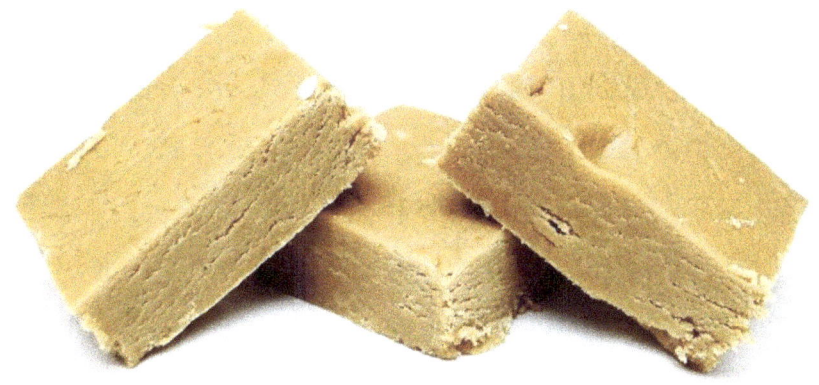

Preparation Time: 10 minutes

Cooking Time: 0 minute

Servings: 12

Ingredients:

- 12 oz smooth peanut butter
- 3 tbsp coconut oil
- 4 tbsp coconut cream

- 15 drops liquid stevia
- Pinch of salt

Directions:

1. Line baking tray with parchment paper.
2. Melt coconut oil in a saucepan over low heat.
3. Add peanut butter, coconut cream, stevia, and salt in a saucepan. Stir well.
4. Pour fudge mixture into the prepared baking tray and place in refrigerator for 1 hour.
5. Cut into pieces and serve.

Nutrition:

Calories 125, Fat 11.3g, Carbohydrates 3.5g Sugar 1.7g, Protein 4.3g, Cholesterol 0mg

NOTE

www.ingramcontent.com/pod-product-compliance
Lightning Source LLC
Chambersburg PA
CBHW072205100526
44589CB00015B/2380